HeLa Cells of Henrietta Lacks

By

Nishi Singh

Disclaimer:

Whilst every care is taken to ensure that the information in this book is as up-to-date and accurate as possible, no responsibility can be taken by the author for any errors or omissions contained herein. Some images used in this book are in the public domain compiled from various image repositories. Research for the book has been done using reliable sources and the author's own person experience. In the event where any fact or material is incorrect or used without proper permission, please contact us so that the oversight can be corrected.

Table of contents

What are HeLa cells?

HeLa cells are not something that too many people know about, unless you have studied the history of modern American medicine. HeLa cells are simply a cell population that was originally derived from a woman in 1951 named Henrietta Lacks, which whom the cells are named after. Henrietta was a cancer patient who had cervical cancer, which is a cancer that originates in the cervix area of the body. However, her cells were found to be quite different than normal human cells. A scientist by the name of George Otto Gey found her cells to have the ability to grow in a culture dish and eventually concluded that they were an immortal cell line. This means the cells would not stop replicating, which allowed Dr. Gey to place the HeLa cell line into cell culture flasks in order to be preserved. Since the cell line is immortal, it was able to survive in an in vitro state and allowed scientists to use the cancer cells in order to experiment with vaccines and medicines.

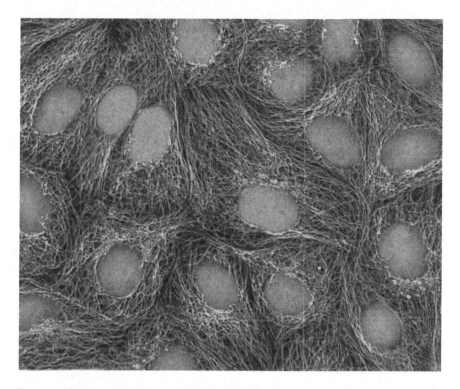

Image of cultured HeLa cells: The Golgi apparatus is shown as orange, microtubules as green and DNA as cyan. Source: National Institutes of Health (NIH)

HeLa cells were the first cell lines to be kept in vitro and it opened up many scientific doors that led towards the miracle of modern medicine. The only controversy that has sprung up regarding these cells has been from the family of Henrietta, particularly her granddaughter Jeri Lacks-Whye. The family is upset that nobody asked for permission for Henrietta cells to be taken and used for scientific research, including Henrietta herself. Not only that scientists have been reluctant to share information with the family regarding any scientific discoveries that have been derived from the HeLa cells.

The cells of Henrietta Lacks were the first cells to ever be captured that replicated themselves. They are also the first human cells to be successfully cloned in 1955. This makes HeLa cells the oldest immortal human cell line in existence that is still being used by doctors and scientists to this day. HeLa cells where the first cells to be sent in space to learn about the effects of zero gravity on human cells. Scientists even developed the famous polio vaccine from them. As medical professionals around the world learned of the successes that American scientists were having with HeLa cells, the global demand for these cells also increased rapidly. The HeLa cells were being grown in mass quantities and shipped off to other scientists around the world. Many of these international scientists wanted to use the cells to research a wide variety of diseases and viruses, such as AIDS, cancer and toxic poisons. But besides all of these life changing pursuits, HeLa cells have also been used for testing products as well. Consumer items, like makeup, tape and glue, have been tested with HeLa cells in order to determine their sensitivity to humans.

As of today, scientists have grown about 40,000 pounds of HeLa cells and have registered over 11,000 patents that involve the use of these cells. With the basically unlimited supply of cells that can be replicated, scientists continue to use HeLa cells as the basis of all their cancer and virus research. By studying how these viruses affect cells, scientists are able to learn of ways to counterattack these affects.

Where did HeLa cells come from?

HeLa cells originally came from a woman named Henrietta Lacks. The name "HeLa" was derived from the first two letters of her first and last name. Henrietta was a woman who was suffering from cancer in the cervix area of her body. What was unique about Henrietta was that her cells that were derived from her cervix would never stop replicating themselves to produce more cells outside her body. This was a medical breakthrough for the scientific community because they could experiment with vaccines and medicines on these cancer cells in order to produce new treatments for people who had similar problems. Since the cells keep replicating, it gives medical researchers endless opportunities to experiment with the cells while kept in vitro. More than 60 years after Henrietta passed away, HeLa cells are still being used by doctors and scientists to this day.

The first time HeLa cells were obtained was when doctors removed pieces of the cancerous tumor that had grown inside Henrietta Lacks' cervix region. The doctors also removed healthy cells for her cervix region as well, so they could be studied for future medical research along with the cancerous cells. The HeLa cells were eventually passed on to other medical researchers, the first being Dr. George Gey of Johns Hopkins University. Dr. Gey was the director of the newly constructed Tissue Culture Laboratory at Johns Hopkins University in the early 1950s. He was also the first one to replicate the cells, so that other scientists and researchers around the world could experiment with them. Now days these cells are replicated at the National Institutes of Health and shipped out to other doctors around the world. It is estimated that over 40,000 pounds of HeLa cells have been produced since 1951.

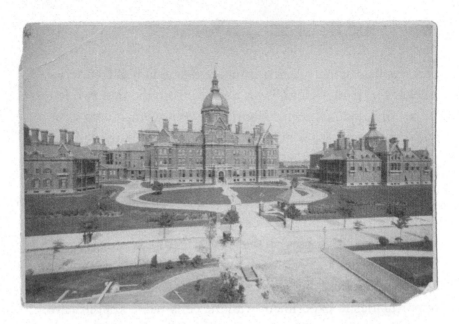

Johns Hopkins Medical Institutions Buildings

What makes HeLa cells so special is the fact that they were the first cells to survive outside the body and that it be can be grown in culture for external examination. Most ordinary cells would stop replicating and would eventually die after a couple of days of being outside their natural biological state. Now you may be wondering why Henrietta's cells were the first to survive in-vitro or outside their biological surroundings. You have to remember that cell culture (science of growing cells) was pretty much in the dark ages before 1950. Scientists knew a little about it, but they never had much chance for experimenting on cells outside of their natural biological state. The reason is because they had simply never discovered a patient who's cells would grow outside the body and therefore cold not establish a cancer cell line. It doesn't mean that one did not exist. It just means that scientists had never discovered one before they examined Henrietta Lacks at Johns Hopkins Hospital in 1951. Once they discovered the type of cells she had, they jumped at the chance to culture them. That is likely the reason why they never asked for permission from Henrietta or her family to take her cellular tissue. After all, if they had refused to give consent then scientists would have lost the opportunity to capture these rare durable cells. So, they took them without consent, which still remains a controversial topic today. On one hand, the actions of the doctors and scientists have helped find treatments that have helped many other people. On the other hand, they were being unethical to the Lacks family. The true answer of what should have happened will always be up for debate.

Who was Henrietta Lacks?

Henrietta Lacks was an African-American woman from Virginia who was born in the year 1920. After her mother died when she was 4-years-old, she went to live with her grandfather in his log cabin. This is where she got to meet and get close to her cousin, David Lacks. The two eventually formed a romantic relationship as they got older. They ended up moving to Maryland with their cousins in order to get work there on a farm. At first, Henrietta was a typical black woman during this time period that worked the crop fields and tried desperately to support their family. In Henrietta's case, she worked the tobacco fields and ended up having five children before the age of 30. Not only did she have five children, but she had them with her own cousin, David Lacks. This might seem out of place and inappropriate in modern times, but back in those days it was not unusual for people in the south to marry and have kids with their cousins. One day when she was 31-years-old, she felt some kind of knot inside her body. Her cousins had told her that she was probably pregnant again, but after she had her fifth child she began to bleed profusely. After she tested negative for syphilis, her doctor eventually sent her to Johns Hopkins Hospital. This was the only hospital in Maryland at the time that would treat black patients.

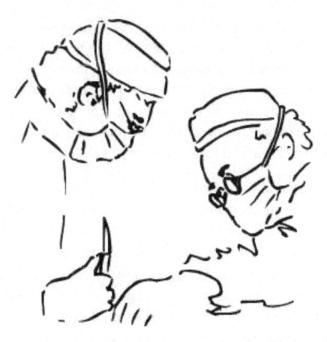

When she when to the hospital, it was discovered that she had a cancerous tumor in her cervix. The doctors at Johns Hopkins treated Henrietta with radium tubes and radiation. However, during one of her radiation treatments the doctors removed pieces of her cervix without her permission. One piece was a healthy part and the other was a cancerous part. These pieces were given to a scientist by the name of George Otto Gey, which was the beginning of the immortal cell line known as "HeLa." In the beginning he kept it a secret by telling everyone that these cells came from a woman called Helen Lane hence HeLa cells. She was soon forgotten but in 1970, she was recognized as the real donor of these cells.

Henrietta Lacks never knew what the doctors had done. As she continued to go to Johns Hopkins Hospital for treatment, there was no improvement in her condition. She continued to have great pain, even after having blood transfusions. In October of 1951, she began to have kidney failure and passed away at the young age of 31-years-old. When the body was autopsied, it was found that the cancer had spread in the entire body. She was buried in an unmarked grave in the family cemetery in Lackstown which is a part of Clover in Halifax County, Virginia. But Dr. Roland Pattillo of Morehouse School of Medicine was kind enough to donate a headstone after he had read Rebecca Skloot's "The Immortal Life of Henrietta Lacks".

For a woman who lived such a short life, she unexpectedly made a great impact on many people's lives. Without her HeLa cells, we wouldn't have as much knowledge about the effects of viruses, such as AIDS, and the possible treatments that can be applied to it. Unfortunately, Henrietta never got to live long enough to see the impact she was going to have on people and the scientific community. She never even knew that her cells were taken when she was alive, so she had no way of knowing while she was alive that her cells would be so revolutionary to the world. It even took her family 20 years after Henrietta's death to finally learn about the impact her cells had. In 2010, there was a book written about Henrietta called, "The Immortal Life of Henrietta Lacks." Oprah Winfrey is also trying to produce a movie based on this book. Fortunately, Henrietta is finally getting the recognition that she so rightful deserves.

Epithelial adenocarcinoma and HeLa

Epithelial adenocarcinoma is the scientific way of describing the cell line of a cancerous tumor that is usually found in animal tissue. In the case of Henrietta Lacks, her HeLa cells are a human version of an epithelial adenocarcinoma. Her cell line was created after Dr. Howard Jones of the Johns Hopkins Hospital had taken a piece of her tumor and had it studied for scientific research purposes. The 31-year-old Henrietta Lacks was already being treated for cervical cancer at the time, but she died in less than a year after being treated.

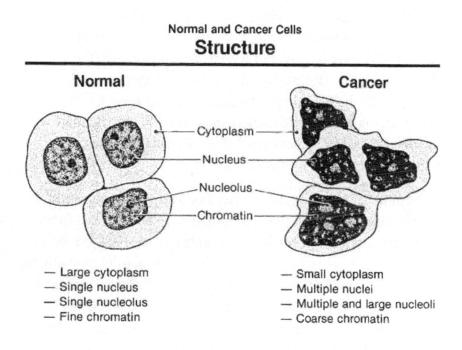

Normal and Cancer Cells
Structure

Normal	Cancer
— Large cytoplasm	— Small cytoplasm
— Single nucleus	— Multiple nuclei
— Single nucleolus	— Multiple and large nucleoli
— Fine chromatin	— Coarse chromatin

No one outside the scientific community usually uses the term "epithelial adenocarcinoma" to describe the HeLa cell line. But when a scientist looks at those words, they know exactly what they mean because they describe the type of cell line it is. The word "epithelial" is another way of describing one of the four types of body tissues. The epithelial tissues align the body cavities with the structures of the body. As for the epithelial cells that make up these tissues, they have the function of protection, absorption, sensation and more. The word "Adenocarcinoma" describes a cancerous tumor that can form in many different parts of the body. So when we say "epithelial adenocarcinoma," we are describing epithelial tissue that is forming a tumor.

In the case of Henrietta Lacks, the abnormalities in her epithelium caused her to get cervical cancer. Radiation treatment was given to her to slow down the spreading of this cancer, but it eventually got the best of her and ended up killing her in October of 1951. When the autopsy was performed on Henrietta, they found that the cancer had successfully spread throughout her entire body. This is danger of having abnormalities in the epithelial region. If the body cavities are not lined properly to the organs of the body because of cancer, then the organs will eventually fail. Henrietta Lacks experienced kidney failure, which was ultimately her cause of death outside of the cancer that was responsible for the failure.

The epithelial adenocarcinoma cell line known as "HeLa cells" are the oldest and most popular human cell line still used in the scientific community. Medical researchers all around the world have received clones of these HeLa cells in order to help with the scientific research process. HeLa cells have become a standard for learning about essential biological processes. Scientists have used the cells for experimenting with the polio vaccine, creating cloning techniques and mastering vitro fertilization. Most importantly, they are learning to identify the cause of cervical cancer. With this knowledge, they are hoping to develop the first ever anti-cancer drug that will totally prevent someone from getting cancer. This drug will only be given to someone who has the very early signs of cervical cancer. Since the HeLa cells derived from a cervical cancerous tumor, then they may very well be the link to diagnosing in its early stages and preventing it from getting to the point where it becomes fatal.

Life of Henrietta

Henrietta Lacks was an African American woman who was born in Roanoke, Virginia on August 1st, 1920. Her original birth name was Loretta Pleasant, but she eventually changed her name to Henrietta Lacks when she got older. As you can imagine, Henrietta had a pretty hard life being a black woman in early 20th century America. On top of that, her mother died in 1924 when Henrietta was only 4-years-old. After her mother died, Henrietta got to live with her grandfather. He resided in a log cabin that was originally built as slave quarters and previously owned by a white ancestor of hers. Besides her grandfather, she lived there with her cousin, David Lacks. As the two grew older, they developed a relationship and had five kids together. Eventually, they got married in 1941 and moved to Maryland after their other cousin insisted on it. She got a job working on a tobacco farm with her other cousins.

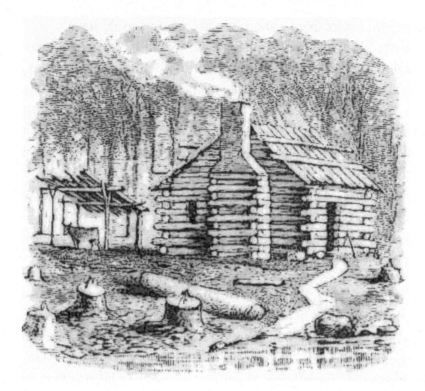

On the day of January 29th, 1951, Henrietta began to feel some unusual pains in her stomach. These pains eventually intensified and she began having abdominal bleeding. Her cousins told her that she was probably pregnant again, but she went to Johns Hopkins Hospital anyways to get a professional diagnosis. At the time, this was the nearest hospital in Maryland that would treat black people. The doctor that examined her, Dr. Howard Jones immediately discovered that she had cervical cancer. The only thing the doctors could do to treat her was give her radiation treatments to slow down the cancer growth. During one of these treatments, doctors took it upon themselves to remove two pieces of her cervical tumor without telling her or any of her family members. Henrietta eventually died on October 4th, 1951. She was only 31-years-old.

Henrietta Lacks lived a short life, but no one could have predicted how much of an impact she would have on many more people's lives. The pieces from Henrietta's tumor were sent to a special research laboratory that was headed by Dr. George Otto Gey. After Dr. Gey examined the cells of the tumor, he noticed how unusual they appeared to be. Most cells can only survive a few days in vitro, but Dr. Gey found that Henrietta's cells were staying alive and divided rapidly. This motivated Dr. Gey to multiply these cells and create a whole new cell line based off of Henrietta's cells. This cell line was given the name "HeLa," which comes from the first two letters of Henrietta's first and last name.

A few years later, the HeLa cell line had already revolutionized the entire medical industry. A medical researcher, Jonas Salk, used the HeLa cells to help create a vaccine for polio. Once this happened, scientists and researchers all around the world were interested in this cell line. Scientists in America began cloning the cells and shipping them to other scientists from around the world. Since 1955, over 11,000 patents have already been registered that involve the use of HeLa cells.

The family of Henrietta Lacks

Anyone that is remotely interested in medical science or research has probably heard of HeLa cells and the person they came from, Henrietta Lacks. But, what do people really know about the family of Henrietta Lacks? The only information that has made any real headlines is the fact that Henrietta's family have complained that nobody, including Henrietta, gave permission for doctors to use her cells. The family didn't even learn about the existence of the cells until 1973, which was over 20 years after the cells were originally taken from Henrietta's cervical tumor. What's worse is the family was not formally notified about the cells. The only reason they were told by scientists was because they needed blood samples and genetic materials from all of Henrietta's living relatives. So obviously, the scientists had to come forward with the truth about their intentions with the HeLa cells in order to get the family to cooperate with donating their genetic material. As you can imagine, this outraged the family and they felt they deserved to know about the HeLa cells when they were first taken from Henrietta back in 1951. When the family tried to make inquiries to the scientists as to the specific use of the HeLa cells, their requests got ignored. The scientists wouldn't even tell them which publications contained their genetic information that was based on the genetic material they had submitted to them.

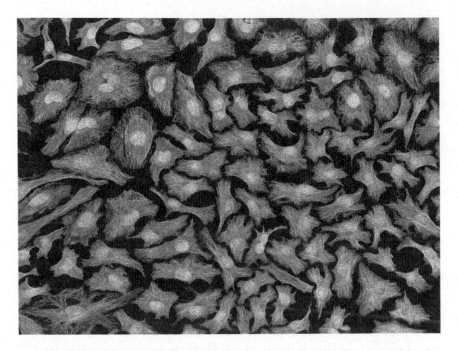

Multiphoton fluorescence image of HeLa cells with cytoskeletal microtubules (magenta) and DNA (cyan). Source: National Institutes of Health (NIH)

The family continued to be kept in the dark over the years until 1998, which was when the British Broadcasting Corporation aired an <u>award-winning documentary about Henrietta Lacks and her HeLa cells</u>. About 10 years later, an author by the name of Rebecca Skloot had written a book about Henrietta called "The Immortal Life of Henrietta Lacks." This book quickly gained a new fan base and it even inspired Oprah Winfrey to make plans to produce a film based on this book. With all of this new attention brought to the Lacks family, the contributions made by Henrietta Lacks and her cells have now been publically recognized. As for the Lacks family, they were honored at the National Foundation for Cancer Research and the Smithsonian Institution. Henrietta Lacks even received a posthumous honorary degree from Morgan State University. As for her unmarked grave, a man by the name of Dr. Roland Pattillo from Morehouse College had generously purchased a headstone to be placed there.

The Lacks family waited almost 60 years to get the public recognition that they and Henrietta deserved. The National Institutes of Health (NIH) located in Bethesda, Maryland, which oversees the HeLa cell line, has even formed an agreement with the Lacks Family to acknowledge them in all scientific papers. They are even giving them power to oversee some of the decisions made with the genome sequence of the cells. Jeri Lacks-Whye, the granddaughter of Henrietta Lacks, is usually the one who represents the voice of the family. She is pleased with the new advancements towards her family's rights; however, she would prefer that they get to oversee all of the decisions made with the HeLa cells, not just the genome sequence.

Dr. George Otto Gey – The man behind HeLa cells

Dr. George Otto Gey is considered to be a pioneer in the medical field of cellular and cancer research. Coincidentally, the man who spent his whole life studying cancer cells had also gotten cancer himself and passed away on November 8th, 1970. While he was alive, he achieved many great things. His first award was his Bachelor of Science degree that was issued by the University of Pittsburgh. After graduating, he got a job as a Zoology instructor at the university for two years. Then in 1923, he began to collaborate with Margaret and Warren Lewis who worked at Johns Hopkins University. Gey was given a job there as the director of the Tissue Culture Laboratory, which was located in the Department of Surgery. This gave him the opportunity to work towards his Doctor of Medicine degree, which he earned in 1933. After that, his career grew very fast. He eventually became the director of the famous Finney-Howell Cancer Research Laboratory in 1947, which was a job he continued until his death in 1970. However, it was at this job that gave him the opportunity to be the first one to experiment with HeLa cells.

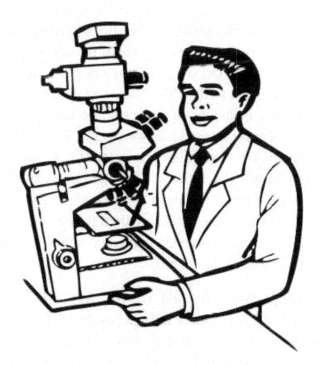

These HeLa cells are tumor cells that were originally extracted from the cancerous cervical tumor of a woman named Henrietta Lacks. She had originally been treated at Johns Hopkins Hospital with radiation therapy, which did little to help stop the cancer from growing throughout her body. However, her main doctor, Dr. Howard Jones, was able to get samples of her cells while she was still alive. He took both healthy cells from the cervix and cancerous cells from the tumor and sent them over to Dr. Gey at his Tissue Culture Laboratory in Johns Hopkins Hospital. Dr. Gey was responsible for replicating the cells into the first immortal cell line to be kept in vitro. In fact, he was able to take one specific cell and grow it in a petri dish using chicken plasma and eventually start a cell line. These cells continued to multiply and grow unlike the previous ones he had tried to establish. He now had the first immortal human cell line which he called the HeLa cells.

Layman people typically know Dr. Gey from his dealings with the HeLa cells. Very few people outside of the scientific community realize that Dr. Gey was also a popular lecturer and sought after consultant in the 1950s. He even received many honorable awards, including the Catherine Berkan Judd Award for his work in Cancer Research as well as the Wien Award for Cancer Cytology. Dr. Gey had been a doctor for 47 years, from 1933 to 1970. Within that time, he developed numerous techniques used in the cell cultures in virology, endocrinology, cytology and oncology. He is also credited for having created the roller drum, which was a machine that could actually nurture various cell cultures while in vitro.

Outside of the professional world, Dr. Gey was an avid fisherman and enjoyed outdoor adventures. In 1970, he ended up dying of pancreatic cancer. Dr. Gey was still a scientist up until the very end because he had asked the doctors to remove a piece of cancer growth from his liver, so a new cell line could be made for further medical research. Unfortunately, the doctors did not oblige and this greatly upset Dr. Gey all the way to his death.

Some consider Dr Gey as someone who took Henrietta's cells for his own good but one has to remember that he was the one who labeled the cells in a way in which he incorporated the first two letters of her names. If he wanted he could have named the cells anything he liked or could have used a random number. It seems as if he honored Henrietta. So every time we think of HeLa cells, we think of Henrietta Lacks. It is true that the staff at Johns Hopkins Hospital should have taken the consent of the family before using the cells but in those days things like patient consent, medical ethics, and privacy did not exist.

How are HeLa cells grown in culture?

If you are not a cell culture scientist then this protocol will be of
little importance to you but nonetheless let's take a look how
HeLa cells can be grown in culture. In fact the protocol below is
used for growing HeLa cells all around the world.

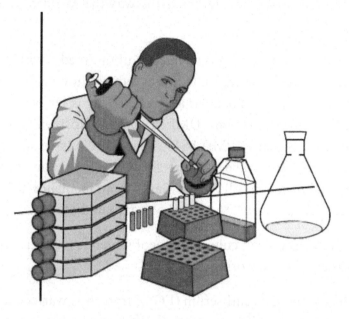

Initially, when the cervical tumor was excised off the cervix of
Henrietta Lacks, it was sent to the lab of Dr Gey. Her technician
cut the tumor in small pieces and plated them out in homemade
cell culture media made from chicken serum, special growth
salts, and placentas and placed them in a roller drum which they
used as an incubator. These roller drums just like a cement roller
was a machine that Dr Gey had invented so that it would slowly
spin twice every hour to mix the substances that were inside. It
had holes that allowed the allocation of appropriate growth
substances to be added to the cells. Dr Gey thought that the
spinning was necessary to replicate the flow of cells, the
nutrients and body fluids just like in a body.

He was right in many ways. The cells today are subjected to an artificial bodily environment for them to grow where they are fed and kept at on optimal condition for them to survive. These days, there are commercially available cell culture media that support the growth and maintenance of cells. For the technician at Dr Gey's lab, it was a routine job for her. But little did she know that those cells will revolutionize the way the world will look at cell culture.

HeLa cells needs to be grown in cell culture media with appropriate nutrients and at the right temperature just like all other cells. The most popular available today is Dulbecco's Modified Eagle's medium (DMEM) and the Roswell Park Memorial Institute (RPMI) 1640. These media have appropriate amounts of mineral and vitamins for the cells to grow. The cells can be incubated in cell culture flasks in an incubator at 37 degree Celsius with 95% air and 5% carbon dioxide.

Here's the HeLa cell culture protocol which is used for growing in labs around the world.

1. The media, fetal calf serum (FCS), trypsin is warmed to 37 degrees Celsius using a water bath. FCS is widely used in cell culture to supplement cells with vitamins, growth factors, hormones and other nutrients to help cells grow and proliferate.

2. The old cell culture media is removed from the cell culture flask and any remaining media is removed by washing it with phosphate buffered saline (PBS). PBS is not toxic to cells and often Ethylenediaminetetraacetic acid (EDTA) is used on cells that are clumped together. Trypsin/EDTA mixture is added to the cells to the cover the surface of the cells and the flask is placed back in the incubator. Trypsin allows the HeLa cells that are stuck to the bottom of the flask to become detached. Remember they are adherent cells meaning that they are stuck to the surface

of the flask. Incubating the cells with trypsin for about 5 minutes at 37 degrees Celsius speeds the detachment process.

3. Some media is added to the cells and then pipetted a few times to remove clusters of cells. The cells are then centrifuged at 1000g. Centrifugation allows the cells to collect at the bottom of the polypropylene tube.

4. The cells are then plated out in fresh media with FCS and then placed in the incubator at at atmosphere of air at 95% and carbon dioxide at 5% at the temperature: of 37°C.

Watch this video to find out more.
http://www.helacells.com/splitting-hela-cells/

Why are HeLa cells immortal?

One of the major differences between a normal somatic (body) cell and a cancer cell is that the cancer cell has the ability to proliferate (divide) indefinitely. This means that cancer cells, either in the body or when cultured in flasks have an unlimited dividing potential, hence are immortal. The age of normal cells are not determined by chronological time but the number of cell division it has gone through. It serves as a kind of age clock that determines how long it has to live by counting the allocated cell divisions it has gone through. But for some reason HeLa cells do not have a limit to the number of cell divisions it can go through and hence it can divide indefinitely. We will look at why this happens?

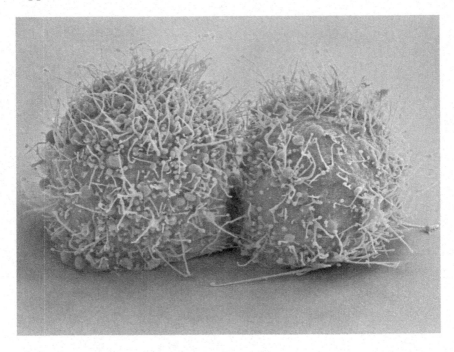

Scanning electron micrograph of divided HeLa cells. Source: National Institutes of Health (NIH)

A phenomenon called the Heyflick limit or Hayflick phenomenon has been suggested to support this. It is thought a normal cell will divide up to 50 to 60 times after which it stops dividing and enters irreversible growth arrest called cell senescence.

Basically the number of times normal cells undergo cell division before it reaches senescence or cell death is called the Heyflick limit. This allows the body to prevent accumulation of faulty cells or cells that have mutations that might become cancerous. Experiments have shown that there is a progressive loss of the telomeric ends of chromosomes called "telomeres" which plays an important timing mechanism in human cellular aging.

The role of the telomeres is to prevent chromosomes from destabilising. Another role is to prevent chromosomes from fusing or merging to each other. They cap the ends of chromosomes with repetitive telomere sequences that protect the ends from damage and rearrangements. However, there is an enzyme called "telomerase" that adds the sequence "TTAGGG" repeats onto mammalian telomeres which prevents their shortening after cell division. One of the first steps of tumorigenesis (formation of cancer) is the activation of telomerase in malignant cells. HeLa cells have the active form of this very enzyme that makes it grow indefinitely.

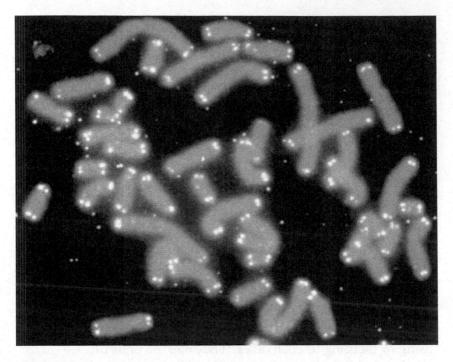

Human chromosomes in grey capped by telomeres in shiny white.
Source: U.S. Department of Energy Human Genome Program

Telomerase are eukaryotic ribonucleoprotein (RNP) complexes that have essential RNA and a protein reverse transcriptase subunit. By using the process of reverse transcriptase, it is able to maintain the length of the telomeres in all cancer cells. In other words, it's a reverse transcriptase enzyme that forms telomeres.

Every time a cell divides, it loses about 25-200 base pairs of DNA till it reaches a length that is called the "critical length" and causes the cell undergo apoptosis or programmed cell death. The enzyme telomerase adds the DNA sequence TTAGGG at the ends of the chromosomes and prevents it from reaching the critical length. There is very little activity of telomerase in normal body cells. However the enzyme is found in fetal tissues, adult germ cells, and cancer cells. HeLa cells have an active form of the telomerase enzyme allowing the cells to maintain its chromosomal length and never reaching that critical length and therefore preventing it from dying and causing them to grow uncontrollably.

Hence, we can classify HeLa cells as "Telomerase-positive human cervical carcinoma" cells line as they have increased telomerase activity. If these telomerases were to be turned off somehow then the telomeres of these cells will also shorten and eventually die.

There is a lot of research going on in the field of telomerase using HeLa cells so that an effective anticancer therapy (anti-cancer therapeutic agents for example telomerase inhibitor) could be devised where human tumors have the active form of telomerase.

HeLa cell controversy

For over 60 years, HeLa cells have allowed medical researchers to experiment with new medications and treatments towards fighting cancer. Everyone in the scientific community is pleased with their results and advancements in modern medicine that have derived from HeLa cells. This is all due to a woman named Henrietta Lacks and her immortal cell line. After she died in 1951, medical researchers took her cells and allowed them to grow for all of these years. However, the family of Henrietta Lacks claims they never gave consent to any of these doctors to take Henrietta's cells and experiment with them. As of today, the National Institutes of Health have claim over HeLa cells. Fortunately, they are trying to compromise with the remaining family members of Henrietta in regards to all the genomic sequential information taken from the HeLa cells. So now, if medical researchers want to access any of the data from this genome sequence then they'll have to get the approval of a medical panel, which includes Henrietta's remaining family members.

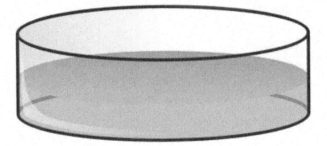

What was truly hard for the Lacks family was that they had to wait 20 years after Henrietta's death to learn that her cells had been kept in vitro. The only reason they found out was because medical scientists wanted to use Henrietta's children in a series of experiments. Later on, the children's medical records were released based on these experiments, even though they had not consented to them being released. As you may know, a patient's medical records and history is supposed to be kept confidential from the public. Therefore, the rights of the Lacks' family had been violated and the controversy between them and the scientists continued on for years afterwards.

You might be wondering why Henrietta's relatives would be so upset about medical researchers using her cells. It's not that they don't want there to be advancements in modern medicine. Her family was simply upset because the doctors never asked permission nor have they shared any of their scientific findings with them. Now that has changed, but only for information pertaining to the genome sequence. Also, the Lacks family is not receiving any kind of financial compensation or monetary gain from this new agreement. But still, this is the most progress they have made over this controversy in the last 60 years. It creates the perfect balance of allowing medical science to take advantage of the HeLa cells while allowing the Lacks' family interests to be protected at the same time. Unfortunately, the European Molecular Biology Laboratory (EMBL) had started a new controversy right after the old one with the National Institutes of Health went away. The EMBL had posted up a HeLa cell line's sequential data to public databases, which can be accessible by anyone. This undermines the privacy rights of the Lacks family all over again. Henrietta Lacks' granddaughter, Jeri Lacks-Whye, is still concerned about her family's privacy rights to this day. Although their rights are slowly becoming established, it will likely take many more years for the Lacks' family to get the final say in all decisions related to the HeLa cells.

HeLa genome data use agreement

Henrietta Lacks was the unexpected carrier this amazing cell line. This was a cell line that was able to keep producing new cells and would not die under in vitro conditions. Before Henrietta died of cervical cancer in 1951, her doctors had removed portions of her cancerous tumor and submitted them to cellular cancer research specialist named Dr. George Gey. In August of 2013, The National Institutes of Health formed a new agreement with the family of Henrietta Lacks to allow them access to genome data taken from her cells. In exchange for sharing data received from the HeLa cells, biomedical researchers now have to get permission by the Lacks family to oversee all the genome sequential data of the HeLa cells. The agreement is one that the Lacks family is comfortable with. After all, they don't want to jeopardize the advancements of medical science and the possible new discoveries that could be made with the HeLa cells. All they ever wanted was to be involved in the process and to be informed about any new data that pertains to those cells. The family is now involved in the policy and decision making that goes into how HeLa cells are used for advancing science and protecting the rights of participants of the research. Therefore, the Lacks family will continue to allow scientific research and progress be made with the use of the HeLa cells as long as they acknowledge publically that Henrietta Lacks is the reason for it.

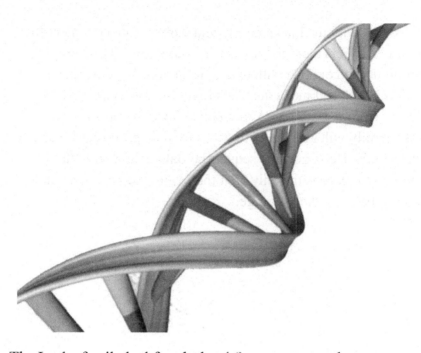

The Lacks family had fought hard for years to get the proper recognition for Henrietta. Unfortunately, their persistence wasn't what started this new agreement between the Lacks family and the National Institutes of Health. It all started when German researchers published their own scientific paper regarding the comparison between healthy human cell tissues and the cell lines from Henrietta, which are the HeLa cells. This scientific paper had some negative reactions from those in the medical industry, from bioethicists to patient advocates and researchers. They claimed it violated the Lacks family's privacy rights. Not only that, the paper mentioned their possible risk of getting disease because of their relation to Henrietta. The Lacks family told German researchers about their worries and concerns over this matter. Fortunately, the German researchers complied and stopped the data of the scientific paper from being accessible by the public. The genome data controversy from this paper brought to light the seriousness of policy and ethical issues regarding the family's rights. So, the medical staff of the National Institutes of

Health met with the Lacks family and came to an agreement that not only respects their privacy issues, but allows the scientific community to continue with using HeLa cells for the greater good of health and medicine. This agreement was entitled the "HeLa Genome Data Use Agreement." Two members of the Lacks family will also get to review any new proposals regarding access to the HeLa genome sequential data. Right now, the genome sequence is the only area they can vote on, but as time goes on that will likely change.

Discoveries made from HeLa cells

HeLa cells are the name given to an immortal cell line that was extracted from Henrietta Lacks' cervical tumor back in 1951. In the 60 years since, there have been quite a number of significant contributions made to modern medicine and science based on the scientific research conducting using those cells. HeLa cells have helped in the development of cancer treatments, vaccines and even in vitro fertilization techniques. Without HeLa cells, we wouldn't have a polio vaccine, chemotherapy, the cancer drug known as "Tamoxifen," gene mapping and treatments towards leukemia, influenza and Parkinson's disease. Many of these treatments are not actually cures, but they help slow down and limit the effects of the symptoms. But besides just medical treatments, HeLa cells have helped in the consumer world as well. Little things, like tape and glue, have been tested using HeLa cells in order to determine how sensitive humans are to them. It is pretty scary to think that we may not have those items if HeLa cells didn't exist. To think, all of this came from one cancer patient in 1951 that happened to have an epithelial cell line that fortunately got discovered by the right doctors. The discoveries that have been made because of HeLa cells have changed modern medicine for the better. The best part is that discoveries and experiments are continuously being made using this cell line.

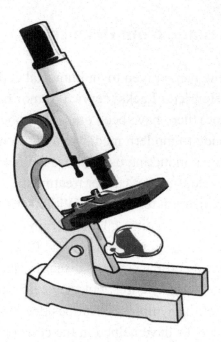

The most popular discovery of them is still the polio vaccine. When Henrietta Lacks died in 1951, this just happened to be around the same time that 10,000 people infected with polio were demanding a cure for their disease. The original polio vaccine was later developed in 1954 by a medical researcher named Jonas Salk. After that, the popularity of the cells within the scientific community took off. The first cell production laboratory, or factory, was built to clone these HeLa cells. The cells also became the first human cells to ever be shipped by the postal service.

As for the future of HeLa cells, they are still serving a hopeful purpose in the scientific community. Medical researchers are hoping to pinpoint the causes of getting cervical cancer and the ways of preventing it from spiraling out of control to the point where it becomes fatal to a person. There are even rumors that anti-cancer drugs will eventually be made from this. Since they basically have an unlimited supply of HeLa cells that they can keep replicating, this means they can keep testing new drugs on the cancer cells and study the reaction it causes to the cell line. This is how all discoveries get made with these cells. The best part is that scientists don't have to worry about damaging or destroying the cells, since they can replicate new ones. After 60 years since this cell line was first obtained, it has already helped treat thousands of patients with various diseases. Once scientists are able to cure cancer with the help of HeLa cells, Henrietta Lacks may very well go down in history as the woman who ultimately was responsible for the cure.

Ethical issues behind the use of HeLa cells

The HeLa cells of Henrietta Lacks have done a lot of good for the scientific and medical communities. However, the ethical dilemma of doctors from Johns Hopkins Hospital taking Henrietta's cells without asking her or her family for permission is still a controversy that exists today. Even though the scientific community has just recently honored Henrietta Lacks and given a little more freedom of information to her family, the ethical use of the cells still remain. Also, HeLa cells have made companies and scientists millions of dollars from selling drugs and human biological matter created through those cells. The Lacks family received none of the profits. This is just one example of why the public does not trust medical research or medical professionals to be honest with them. They are afraid that their medical records won't remain private or that the information in them will be shared with people who are not family members. In the case of Henrietta Lacks, the book "The Immortal Life of Henrietta Lacks" raises public awareness about the unethical behavior of the health industry.

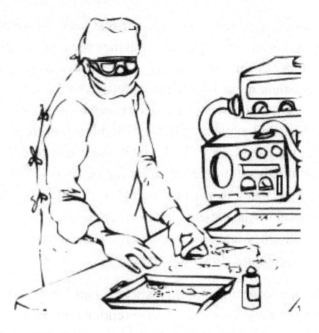

If anything ethically good came out of the Henrietta case, it was that Johns Hopkins Hospital now requires doctors to get consent from their patients before removing their cellular tissue. The patients have to sign a form to give this consent before the surgical procedure is actually performed. Basically, the patients are giving permission for the doctors at Johns Hopkins Hospital to either dispose the tissue or preserve it for educational purposes. If the doctors want to use the tissue for the purposes of scientific research, then the patient's name must be disclosed. However, consent is still more complicated than just having a patient read a contract and then having them sign it. There are some cases in which the patient will have to provide a biospecimen, like blood or DNA, in order to accommodate a unique research project that needs approval from the review board. Most often, the tissue specimens taken from patients are used at an undetermined date in the future.

People are often quick to determine that doctors don't want to get consent because they only care about their own research and making money. You have to remember that patients are not doctors and they do not understand science the way doctors do. When doctors ask for "informed consent" from a patient, this means the patient must understand exactly what their tissues will be used for. Unfortunately, scientific research can be a very complex thing and explaining these difficult scientific terms to layman people is no easy task. So, many doctors and scientists simply feel it is better to not say anything because they don't want to put too many words in general terms and then have it be misunderstood by the patients later on. Therefore, this problem of science illiteracy amongst patients prevents scientists from wanting to communicate with patients.

In the end, however, it is not the patient's fault because their doctors have a duty to explain their intentions properly. This is the ethical thing to do and will increase the amount of trust that people have with their medical professionals.

About the book "The Immortal Life of Henrietta Lacks"

Rebecca Skloot's "The Immortal Life of Henrietta Lacks" is a nonfictional book that tells the life story of Henrietta Lacks and introduces us to her family as well. The book was written to honor the Lacks family and to make the public aware of how much Henrietta Lacks truly contributed to modern science. It tells the story of an African American woman, Henrietta Lacks, who grew up in the racist south of America before 1950. Back then, black women had very few choices for work and so they worked the farm fields to support their families. In Henrietta's case, she worked the tobacco farms with her cousins in Maryland. In 1951, Henrietta was feeling pains in her stomach and went to Johns Hopkins Hospital to seek help, since that was the only hospital in the area that would treat a black woman in those days. She found out that she actually had cervical cancer. The doctors there gave her radiation treatments, but they only postponed the inevitable. However, doctors there cut pieces of her cancerous tumor and sent them to be examined by a medical researcher named Dr. George Gey. He determined these were an immortal cell line that could be replicated over and over again. The book goes into this and the aftermath that these cells had on the world, which became known as "HeLa cells."

It is important to note that this is not a retelling of the story that uses false names or fictionalized elements to enhance the storytelling. All of the names and events that are described in this book are 100% real. The author did extensive research into Henrietta's background. We learn about her years working on the tobacco farm and how she married her cousin, David Lacks. The book does not try to pull any punches. It gives the reader an accurate account of what life was like for Henrietta in those days.

It even goes so far as to recreate scenes from her life along with the dialogue that was said. Skloot spent over a thousand hours interviewing the friends and family of Henrietta as well as various other people connected to the HeLa cell story, including journalists, lawyers, scientists and ethicists. All of this was done by the author to tell the most realistic account of Henrietta's life that was ever told. No one else has even come close to telling Henrietta's story as truthfully and factually as Skloot. The stories of Henrietta before and after her death are both interesting in their own way.

Henrietta could have just been like countless other black women who remained unknown and had no significant story to tell about their lives. In Henrietta's case, she was significant in life and in death. As for her family, they have fought for decades for her privacy rights. With all the popularity of this book, it has opened up new doors for the family. They now have agreements with the National Institutes of Health to have privacy rights and decisions regarding the genome sequential data of the HeLa cells. If it weren't for Skloot's book, this may never have been possible.

Review of "The Immortal Life of Henrietta Lacks" by Rebecca Skloot

The book entitled "The Immortal Life of Henrietta Lacks" gave the long deserved recognition to Henrietta Lacks, who was unintentionally responsible for providing doctors and the scientific community with her miraculous cells which is called the "HeLa Cells." These are durable cell lines that are basically immortal because they can keep replicating into more cells. Not only does this book talk about Henrietta's life, but it also teaches about scientific terms and procedures that most layman people don't know about. But, it is important they have at least some grasp about cells and cell lines because we all have cells. As for Henrietta's cell line, they contributed towards the discovery of many medicines and vaccines which are commonly used today.

The author, Rebecca Skloot, has clearly demonstrated her talents as a writer. Not only that, it is clear that she did her research into Henrietta's life. Skloot takes the reader on an incredible journey throughout the entire life of Henrietta, not just the time she spent at Johns Hopkins Hospital that got her unintentionally famous. That is what is great about this book because it is not just about HeLa cells and the controversy surrounding her family's privacy rights. Skloot has actually written a well told biography about Henrietta Lacks. We got to learn about her work on the tobacco fields and how it was hard for a black woman in the pre-1950 era to find any kind of opportunities.

When you are done reading this book, you will realize that it is a book about family and discovery more than anything else. Since Henrietta Lacks died at the young age of 31, her kids never really got to know their mother. This is especially true for her youngest daughter, Deborah Lacks, who this book focuses on as well. Deborah has been on a journey to learn about her mother all her life. Even though Deborah never knew her mother, she was still inspired by her and even dreamt about being a scientist in her honor. It is clear that Skloot and Deborah collaborated on this book because they both seemed to be on a quest for answers about Henrietta's past. This quest brought them to the real locations of where Henrietta resided, from the tiny tobacco farm in Virginia to her last days at Johns Hopkins Hospital. The book even introduces the reader to the Lacks' family, who are still currently living in Baltimore, Maryland.

The main irony we learn in this book is that Henrietta's family never had health insurance to care for their diseases, but yet Henrietta's immortal cell line has helped treat and cure other people with diseases. The worst part is that the family has not received any monetary compensation on the matter. They only just recently received public recognition, but I hardly think that makes up for all the decades that they were left in the dirt. This book certainly is memorable and I am happy that Oprah Winfrey wants to produce a movie based on this book because it is well deserved. I recommend anyone who likes a heartwarming story to read "The Immortal Life of Henrietta Lacks."

Summary and characteristics of the HeLa cell line

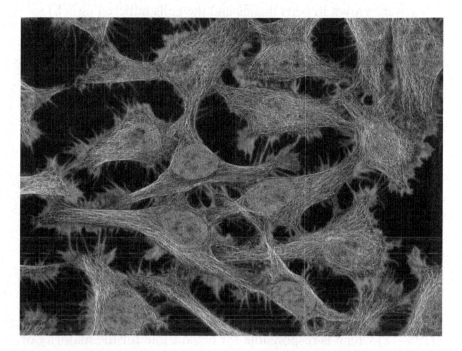

Multiphoton fluorescence image of HeLa cells: Stained with the actin binding toxin phalloidin (red), microtubules (cyan) and cell nuclei (blue). Source: National Institutes of Health (NIH)

HeLa cells are dividing cancer cells that were derived from the cervix of a 31 year old black woman called Henrietta Lacks on 8th February in 1951 at Johns Hopkins Hospital.

In the beginning, "Helen Lane" or "Helen Larson" was named as the source of these cells.

Dr. Howard Jones was her doctor who had examined Henrietta's lump in her cervix.

The biopsy removed from Henrietta was sent to the lab of George Otto Gey without her consent.

George Otto Gey was the scientist who first grew the HeLa cells in culture.

They were grown in petri dishes and the cells adhered (stuck) to the walls of the dishes.

HeLa cells was first human epithelial adenocarcinoma cell line.

They are called immortal because they don't die outside the body and can be grown in vitro.

Hela cells have become the oldest cell line in the world.

The tissue from which HeLa cells originated is the cervix.

These were the first cells to be grown in large quantities.

The HeLa cells were first human cells to be cloned in 1955 by Theodore Puck and Philip Marcus at the University of Colorado.

They are reported to contain the human papilloma virus 18 (HPV-18) which is responsible for responsible for the majority of HPV caused cancers.

They are about 20 microns diameter.

Jonas Salk used these cells to develop a vaccine for polio.

The cells have been used to test human toxicity for tapes, cosmetics, radiation and other toxic substances.

There are about 11,000 patents that involve HeLa cells.

More than 80000 scientific articles had been published from research done on HeLa cells. Just type in "HeLa Cells" in Pubmed and see for yourself.

They are able to divide because these cells have an active version of the enzyme called "telomerase" the enzyme that maintains telomeres (the ends of chromosomes). This prevents HeLa cells from dying.

HeLa cells are difficult to control and have the ability to contaminate other cell cultures.

Most cells are bound by Heyflick limit which is the number of times it can divide after which cell division stops. The HeLa cell can bypass this limit.

Most cancer cells do not have a Heyflick limit.

The complete genome of the HeLa cells was published without the knowledge of the Lacks family in 2013 but when protested, the sequence was withheld from public access.

A data-access committee was set up to make sure that researchers using HeLa cells abide by terms of the HeLa Genome Data Use Agreement of which two members of the Lacks Family are members.

Timeline in the life of the HeLa cell

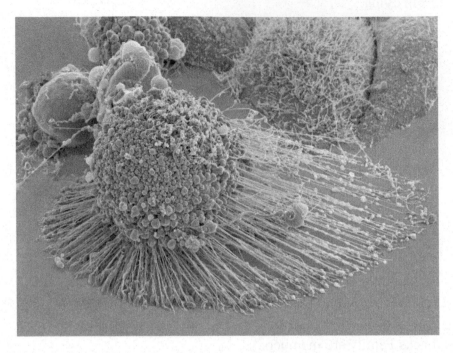

Scanning electron micrograph of a HeLa cell undergoing apoptosis. *Some HeLa cells do undergo apoptosis. Source: National Institutes of Health (NIH)

1951

HeLa cells collected and cultured from the cervix of Henrietta Lacks.

1952

First cells to be posted via mail.

Helped to develop polio vaccine by Jonas Sacks.

Chester M. Southam injects prisoners at the Ohio State Prison with HeLa cells to see if they developed cancer. Half of these prisoners were black.

1953

HeLa cells were stained to show its chromosomes by haematoxylin stain.

1954

First cells to be cloned.

Mass produced for commercial purposes by Microbiological Associates.

1960

First cells to be sent to space to check the effects of human cells in space.

1961

Heyflick limit or number is discovered at about 50.

1965

HeLa is fused with a mouse cell to create the first hybrid cell.

1966

Reports of cultured cells contaminated with HeLa cells begin to appear.

1971

First time HeLa cells are credited to Henrietta Lacks.

1984

HeLa cells are used to show that Human papillomavirus (HPV) is the cause of developing particular types of cancer.

1989

Discovered that HeLa contains the active form of telomerase that causes it to proliferate indefinitely.

1985

Medical records of the family of Henrietta Lacks is published without permission.

1986

HeLa cells are infected with HIV virus to study the virus infection mechanism.

1973

Used to study the effect of salmonella in humans.

2005

HeLa cells are used for Nanotechnology research.

References and further reading

Puck TT, Marcus PI. 1955. A Rapid Method for Viable Cell Titration and Clone Production With Hela Cells In Tissue Culture: The Use of X-Irradiated Cells to Supply Conditioning Factors. Proc Natl Acad Sci USA. 15;41(7): 432-7

Hanks JH, Bang FB. 1917. Dr. George Otto Gey 1899-1970. In Vitro: 6(4): 3-4

The George O. Gey Collection:
http://www.medicalarchives.jhmi.edu/papers/gey.html

Gey GO, et al. 1952. Tissue culture studies of the proliferative capacity of cervical carcinoma and normal epithelium. Cancer Res. 12: 264-265

Lucey BP, Nelson-Rees WA, Hutchins GM. 2009. Henrietta Lacks, HeLa cells, and cell culture contamination. Arch Pathol Lab Med. 133(9): 1463 -7

The HeLa Genome: An Agreement on Privacy and Access - http://www.nih.gov/about/director/statement-hela-08072013.htm

Hudson KL, Collins FS. 2013. Biospecimen policy: Family matters. Nature 500: 141-142

"The Way of All Flesh" BBC documentary - http://www.helacells.com/bbc-hela-documentary

Landry JJ et al. 2013. The Genomic and Transcriptomic Landscape of a HeLa Cell Line. G3 (Bethesda): 3(8): 1213-24

Hanks JH, Bang FB. 1971. Obituary: Dr. George Otto Gey 1899–1970. Cancer Res: 31: 6(4):3-4

Callaway E. 2013. Deal done over HeLa cell line: Family of Henrietta Lacks agrees to release of genomic data. Nature. 07 August 2013

EMBL Press Release: Havoc in biology's most-used human cell line. Genome of HeLa cells sequenced for the first time. Heidelberg, 11 March 2013

Landry JJ et al 2013. The genomic and transcriptomic landscape of a HeLa cell line. G3 Journal. 3: 1213-1224

HeLa Genome Data Use Agreement. August 6, 2013. The National Institutes of Health

Jones HW Jr. 1997. Record of the first physician to see Henrietta Lacks at the Johns Hopkins Hospital: history of the beginning of the HeLa cell line. Am J Obstet Gynecol. 176(6): S227-8

Ncayiyana DJ. 2011. The extraordinary story of the life after death of Henrietta Lacks. S Afr Med J. 101(3): 141

The Immortal Life of Henrietta Lacks by Rebecca Skloot. March 8, 2011

A Conspiracy of Cells: One Woman's Immortal Legacy and the Medical Scandal It Caused by Michael Gold. January 1, 1986

Finding Henrietta Lacks by Michael Rogers. July 24, 2011

Cells For Kids (Science Book For Children) by Nishi Singh

Nakashima M, Nandakumar J, Sullivan KD, Espinosa JM, Cech TR. 2013. Inhibition of telomerase recruitment and cancer cell death. J Biol Chem. 288 (46): 33171-80

Greely HT, Cho MK. 2013. The Henrietta Lacks legacy grows. EMBO Rep. 14(10): 849

Buseh AG1, Stevens PE, Millon-Underwood S, Townsend L, Kelber ST. 2013. Community leaders' perspectives on engaging African Americans in biobanks and other human genetics initiatives. J Community Genet. 4(4): 483 -94

Njoku DB. 2013. The immortal life of Henrietta Lacks. Anesth Analg. 117(1): 286

CPSIA information can be obtained
at www.ICGtesting.com
Printed in the USA
LVOW13s1700011117

554603LV00029B/641/P